MAKE MENTAL GAINS

12 WAYS TO CREATE A FORMULA FOR SUCCESS
IN YOUR BELIEF SYSTEM, LIFE AND BUSINESS

AMY WILHELMI

MAKE MENTAL GAINS

© Copyright 2022, Amy Wilhelmi

No portion of this book may be reproduced by mechanical, photographic or electronic process, nor may it be stored in a retrieval system, transmitted in any form or otherwise be copied for public use or private use without written permission of the Copyright Owner.

It is sold with the understanding that the publisher and the individual authors are not engaged in the rendering of psychological, legal, accounting or other professional advice. The content and views in each chapter are the sole expression and opinion of its author and not necessarily the views of Fig Factor Media, LLC.

For more information, contact:
Amy Wilhelmi | www.amywilhelmi.com
Fig Factor Media, LLC | www.figfactormedia.com

Book Layout by Juan Pablo Ruiz
Printed in the United States of America

ISBN: 978-1-957058-30-6

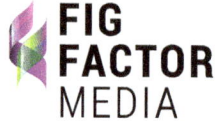

DEDICATION

This book is dedicated to anyone who's ever "been there," fighting through the depths of indecision, the grind of the day-to-day, feeling abnormal, or asking, "Why can't I just be happy?" Perhaps you've tried and failed many times. Maybe you feel like a hamster on a wheel or ask, "Why does everyone around me seem to have their life together, is ambitious, goal-oriented, and passionate, and I just can't seem to catch a break?"

I'm here for you because I've been there, and I've fought my way out of it by developing lifestyle habits that align and have taken me in the direction I want to go. It takes time, consistency, grace, forgiveness, and patience, but you can change your habits, change your mind, change your health, and change your life.

ACKNOWLEDGMENTS

I want to dedicate this book to my family, specifically my husband, children, parents, and friends who have stuck by me through each version of myself that I needed to experience in order to get where I am today. It wasn't always pretty. It probably wasn't always easy to witness as I struggled through various parts of life, but I am loved, and so are you. I am forgiven, and so are you. I walk without shame or judgment with my head held high, for I have been in the depths, and I wish the best for you, too. You can do this. You've got this. I believe in you.

CONTENTS

Introduction 6
Part 1: Belief System 8
    Apathy 11
    Awakening 13
    Ascension 15
    Abundance 17
Part 2: Life 18
    Pillars of Health 21
    Your Body is Your Temple 23
    Value Your Time 25
    Create the Life You Deserve 27
Part 3: Business 28
    Your Team Matters 31
    Delegate and Execute 33
    Relationships, Relationships, Relationships 35
    Keep Your Eyes on The Prize 37
Manifesto 38
About The Author 39

INTRODUCTION

I have evolved. I am on a growth trajectory, and so are you. We are constantly changing and evolving, and that is not without pain or discomfort. Oftentimes in life, we choose the "easier path." We take shortcuts. We give up before we give it time to come to fruition.

The lifestyle habits mentioned in this book did not happen overnight. This was a learning process that took many decades of time to unwind previously held beliefs, identities, family of origin, and attachment issues. I had to go through some very difficult life lessons to be where I am today. I had to take full responsibility for my actions and stop making excuses.

People hate the word obedience, but I had to do just that--be obedient to my core self. I had to shed worrying about what people thought about me for being myself because the truth is, if people don't like you, they aren't your people. There are a million other people in the world that will love you for you.

I had to learn to trust my core self, passions, and life's direction, push through the hard times, prioritize self-care, shed old identities that no longer served me, and make tiny decisions every day that aligned with who I really am--over and over again. I had to ask myself the question, "Is this getting me closer to my dream of abundant living or farther away?" I had to have a complete lifestyle overhaul, letting go of toxic behaviors and heal, leaving no stone unturned. I had to surrender to my destiny.

Being who you are and who you are meant to be, without apology, is the most powerful thing you can do. You have to surrender to being your full and authentic self and, as I say, "Fly your flag." And when you achieve this, the law of attraction brings the resources into your life that you need to fly.

PART 1

BELIEF SYSTEM

It all begins with our mind, our beliefs, and our attitudes.

As a mental health professional, I know how important and crucial mindset truly is. Our belief system is the catalyst for thriving or drowning. Simply put, improving your life begins with YOU.

Leveling up starts with a change of thought, mentality, and mindset followed by BRAVE action.

What does it mean to level up?

It's looking within and finding your WHY, finding what makes you tick, and your reasons for doing what you're doing. It's about introspection and creating your own belief system that will serve you and help to create the life you want. It all starts with understanding four simple words. These four words are a map, the path to your North Star, your journey without even knowing you're on a journey. Hell, you're not even packed or ready to go, but that's life. We are catapulted forward without warning, like leaves in the wind.

The simple truth is we all walk the path of these four words, but we don't always see it at the time.

DON'T FAKE BEING OKAY.
YOU ONLY HURT YOURSELF.
BE REAL WITH WHAT YOU ARE GOING THROUGH.
JUST DON'T LET IT CONSUME YOU.

APATHY

ap·a·thy
noun
Lack of interest, enthusiasm, or concern.

Ever feel like everything is gray and blah? Maybe things that USED to make you feel happy just don't anymore, or you're no longer motivated to achieve your goals? I get it.

Do you feel like you've TRIED to get ahead but exhausted all of your options?

You've tried screaming, mediating, joined a group, negotiated, bought a course, and read ALL the books, yet your motivation to live the life of your dreams seems unattainable. You feel like a hamster on a wheel, and every day is spent on repeat. I get it.

I am here to tell you that this is the first step—KNOWING that you are in this place of apathy. Acknowledging where you are. Being Introspective, owning your suffering in your own mind, and knowing you're not well. Admitting the "stuckness." Personal wellness matters. You can't drive a car on an empty tank. So, let's help fill you up!

WHEN YOU'VE LIVED IN A WORLD OF FEELING CONFIDENT, COMPLETELY YOURSELF, WHOLE, UNBOTHERED BY OTHERS OPINIONS OF YOU.

WHEN YOU SLEEP WELL, EAT WELL, AREN'T STRESSED MOST OF THE TIME, & YOUR BODY IS WORKING WELL, IT'S NOT DESIRABLE TO GO BACK TO WHERE YOU LIVED BEFORE.

AMY WILHELMI, LMFT

AWAKENING

a·wak·en·ing
noun
An act or moment of becoming suddenly aware of something.

Ever learn a fact or piece of information that was so profound and impactful you cannot remember what your life was like before? Did you wake up from the regular view and see it from a whole new perspective? Yeah, I get that. It can be life-changing. It can also be very scary because there's no unseeing it, and there's no going back. Once you've gotten a taste of what life can be like on the other side, you can't stick with vanilla. Well, you can, but you may be pretty miserable.

When you finally realize that you want to take the reins and not live on autopilot anymore, life gets interesting. You begin to have challenging thoughts about the ways that you were living your life. (Cue the reorganization of VALUES, TIME, and PRIORITIES.) You know what life was like before. You know you don't want to be there anymore. So, it's time to make moves. You may change social groups, lose friends, and do things that others view as erratic or selfish. People may say, *"You're not being yourself!"* Good, because you're starting to break out of the mold. You are starting to choose YOU!

Give yourself permission to live a *big life*. Step into who you are *meant to be*. Stop playing *small*. You're meant for *greater things*.

ASCENSION

as·cen·sion

noun

The act of rising to an important position or a higher level.

Every choice you make in your day affects your Optimal Performance. *Every single one*. Your day is a series of choices. If you choose the harder path—the things you DON'T want to do but you HAVE to do—the likelihood of winning your day is HIGHER. If you do this consistently over time, the things you don't want to do simply become the things that you DO want to do. You begin doing them naturally, and they don't feel burdensome anymore. It's the science of habit making--at first new habits seem hard until they seem normal.

As you ascend, you let go of negative coping mechanisms or whatever hinders your growth. This could include hanging out with people who aren't good for you, negative behavior patterns like drinking or smoking, and letting go or not taking care of yourself first.

Community matters. Surround yourself with like-minded people that are on an Ascension Journey who also believe in health and growth—it's the secret sauce. Who you hang out with matters. You need a tribe to hold you accountable and inspire you. You begin to believe that your time is precious, and it is limited only to people who vibe with your energy. You will no longer be tolerant of negativity or drama that brings you down. Your job is to learn from people that are smarter than you—those who have already carved the path you are on today. Ask for help. Take feedback. Then use that feedback and a continual learning process to improve.

our mindset can either propel us forward into our dream life & keep us in a state of happiness + gratitude

OR

it can keep us in negativity & a paralyzed state of spinning our wheels.

the choice is yours

ABUNDANCE

---

a·bun·dance

noun

The state or condition of having a copious quantity of something; plentifulness of the good things of life; prosperity

I believe in the trifecta. When you are truly aligned in your body, brain, and your life's work, you WILL be successful at anything you pursue. It's that simple. Anyone can achieve it if they learn how to let go of old life patterns, unlock, nurture, and then stand in the discipline and consistency to maintain them.

We create and carve a path to abundance in our lives. It's all about your mind. What do you *believe* about your abilities, strengths, and weaknesses? How motivated are you to be on a constant path of improvement? Do you have the mental stamina to stick with it when it gets HARD?

Be patient and think abundantly. It takes time to change your life. When I cut out alcohol from my life, it took me about six months to feel better. I'm a bodybuilder—this takes TIME. There are NO SHORTCUTS. It requires consistency day after day. My training and nutrition plan must be followed to a T to get my desired results. That's it.

There are no gimmicks or shortcuts. It's much simpler than gimmicks or shortcuts, but people don't want simple because simple takes time and planning. Planning matters. I plan my days extensively--my schedule, my kids' schedules—I put my wellness activities on my calendar, and they're non-negotiable. You, too, can have an abundance of time, gratitude, wellness, and more. It's all up to YOU. Choose abundance.

PART 2

LIFE

I am constantly asked, "How do you do it all?"

After all, I am a mom of five, a wife, a mental health therapist, a divorce mediator, an entrepreneur, a bikini bodybuilder athlete, a mindset, business, and growth coach, a speaker, an author, and a changemaker.

My secret is choosing ME. You have to let go of the voices that tell you prioritizing your hopes, dreams, and ambitions is selfish. I've created a framework that works for me and my life.

I teach people how to thrive in their businesses and their lives. How to do it all while living a healthy, mindful, and balanced lifestyle. How to live the lifestyle you're dreaming of--not just dreaming about it, but making it HAPPEN.

You may ask yourself, "When do I start making choices that align with my goals and dreams?"
The answer is that these choices are made in time management, goal setting, strategic planning, relationship, and lifestyle choices.

When will you start choosing YOU?

"THE GOAL IS NOT TO CHANGE WHO YOU ARE, BUT TO BECOME MORE OF WHO YOU ARE AT YOUR VERY BEST."

PILLARS OF HEALTH

Western medicine ignores the wealth of the mind and body connection. It cuts off our heads from our bodies. If you're treating your body like garbage—not getting enough sleep, filling your brain with useless and time-sucking activities, not eating healthy, drinking too much, or not exercising—you're simply not ALLOWING yourself to operate at full capacity or flow.

Prioritize Your Pillars of Health:
- Sleep
- Hydration
- Vitamins and Minerals
- Hormonal Balance
- Nutrition
- Exercise
- Sunlight
- Nature
- Growth Mindset
- Community
- Consistency

Flow only happens when you SURRENDER and deliberately choose the path of alignment. Prioritize your pillars, and you will see how they can truly change your life.

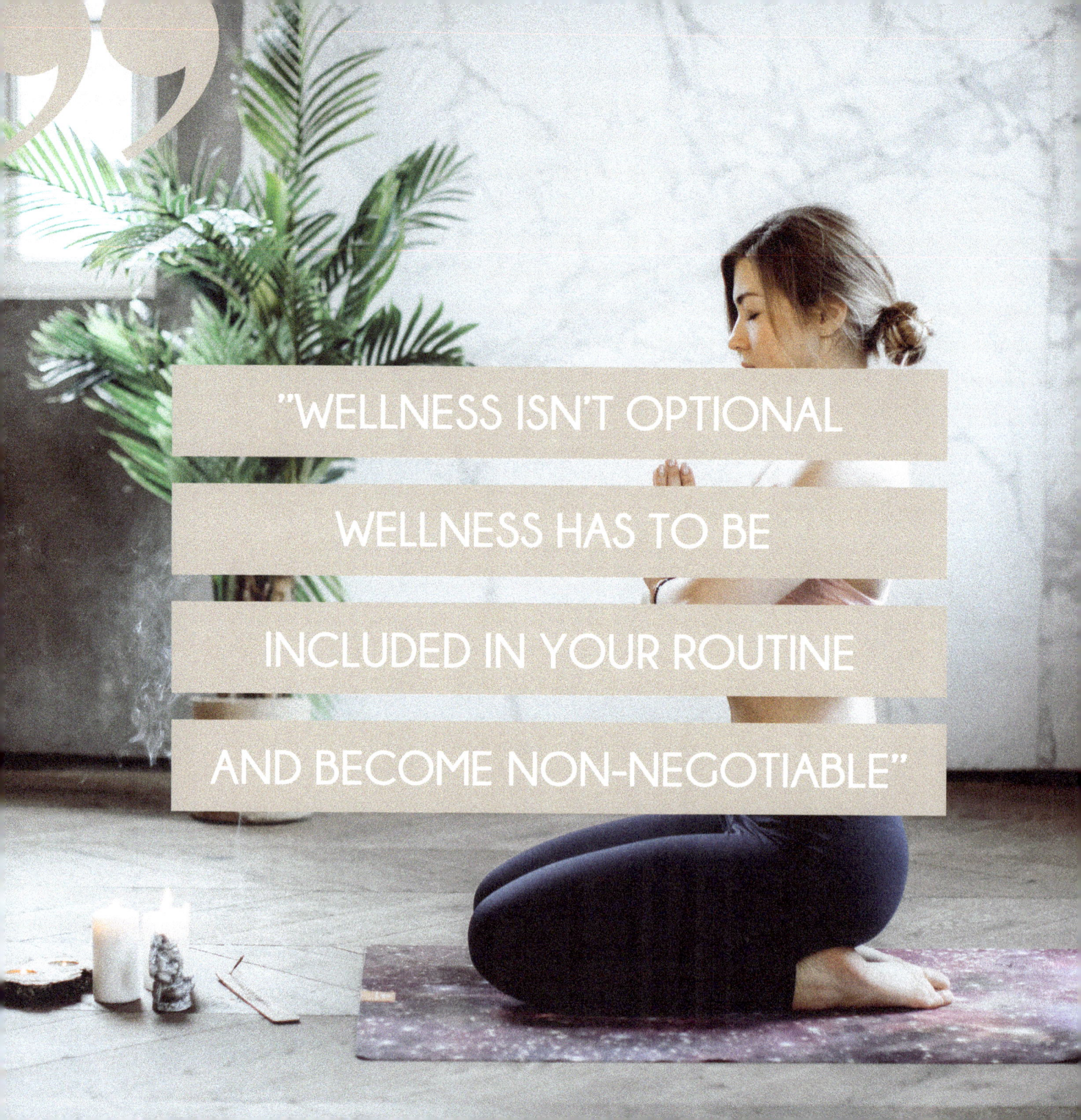

YOUR BODY IS YOUR TEMPLE

As an athlete and bikini bodybuilder, I need to be disciplined to crush my goals. My body demands correct nutrition, calls for needed rest and yearns to build strength. I know my body, and I give it what it deserves. We only have one body, and we either build it or break it.

For me, it looks like this:
- I'm part of the early morning crew and wake up at 4:45 a.m. on days when I don't see my kids off to school.
- My training schedule varies depending on the season, but when I'm not in the gym (usually 5-6 days per week), I'm practicing "active rest," which includes yoga, walking, going out into nature, etc.
- I lift 5-6 days per week, have 3-6 cardio days, in addition to lifting, and then I do yoga.
- I drink a gallon of water and stay hydrated.
- I eat my macros, plan out what I eat every day, and track it. I don't like guessing.
- I go to my chiropractor for care, get a massage every two weeks, and do acupuncture.
- I get my hormones checked and take natural hormone supplements accordingly.
- I know I need nature to recharge, and I take that seriously.
- I take supplements daily, including Vitamin D, Omega 3, a probiotic, and a women's multivitamin.
- I go to bed by 10:00 p.m. and get 6.5 hours of sleep.

If people looked at sleep, nutrition, exercise, nature (unplugging), water intake, early morning routines, massage, chiropractic care, and hormone health as ESSENTIAL to their bodies, life, and work, their lives would absolutely change. What you put into your body matters for your mind.

VIEW YOUR ENERGY AS CURRENCY.

Spend it well.

Invest it well.

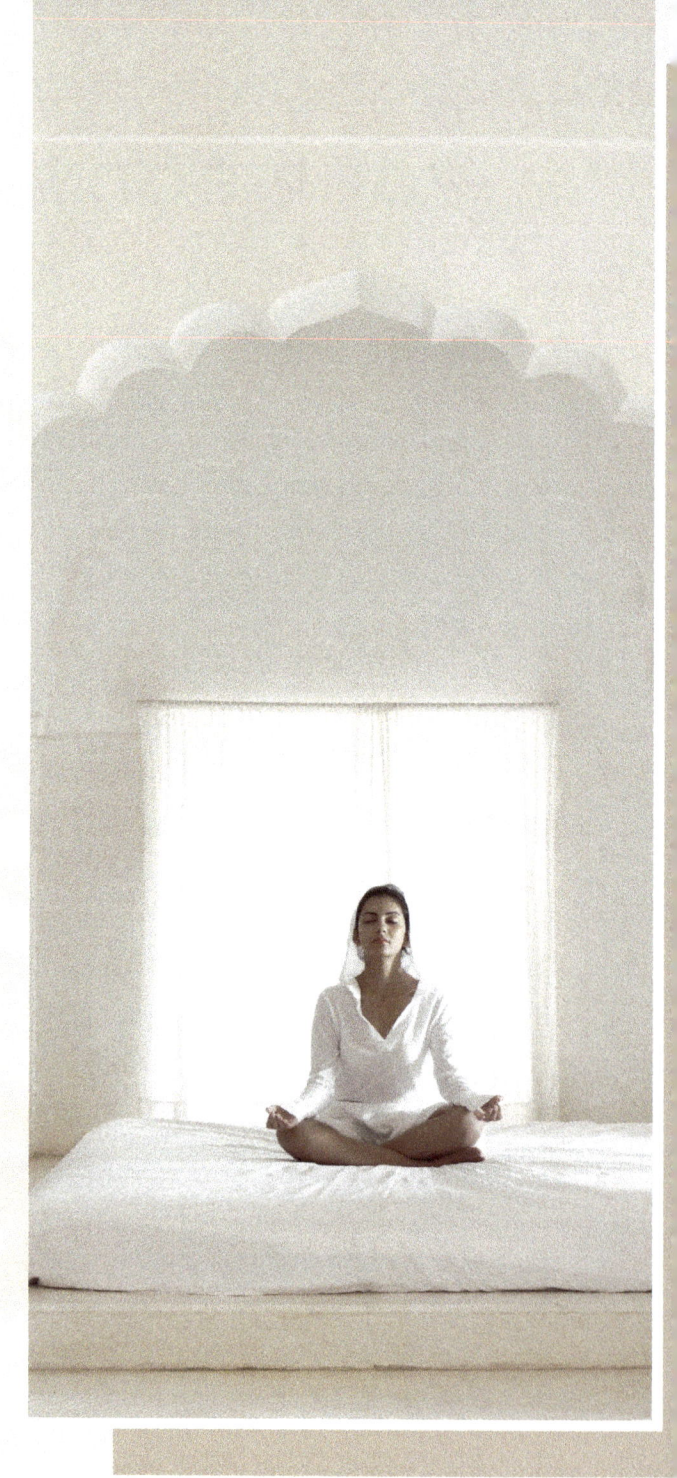

VALUE YOUR TIME

Time is of the essence—a commonly used phrase that holds so much power. For me, my days are strategically planned. Direct client days are limited to two days per week, and then I have the rest of my days for creative pursuits that feed my soul, such as writing, designing, or creating content. So many leaders get burnt out, and startups fail. Why? Because people work themselves to death and DO NOT take care of the essentials.

I value my time—time for myself and time for my family. I'm very protective of my time and, specifically, WHO I give energy to. Those moments that I intentionally carve for myself and my loved ones are essential to my well-being. You need to choose and protect your time, too, so you have time to do what you love.

I practice what I preach. If I'm asking someone else to level up, I'd better be climbing that mountain as well. My clients meet me on my journey, and then we develop a plan to improve their well-being as a team. Strong boundaries are essential, and time is a tool we use to get you there. You need strong time management skills in order to set your priorities. We only have so many hours in the day. Choose wisely.

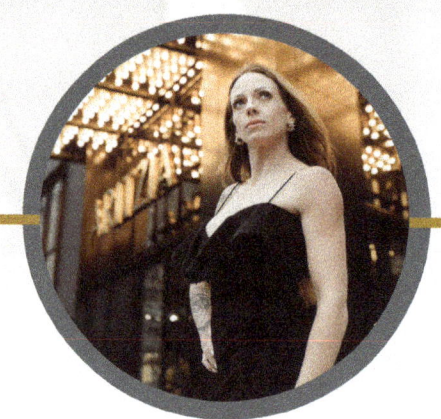

Daily Affirmations

READY? REPEAT AFTER ME.

Success comes with patience.
I am abundant in all the areas of my life.
I am in the right place at the right time,
doing the right thing.
Conscious breathing is my anchor.
I choose to be happy.
I learn by trying new things.

CREATE THE LIFE YOU DESIRE

Working SMARTER, not HARDER, is the way to success. It's the LONG GAME. I am a believer that how you do one thing is how you should be operating in all realms. It's easy to want to take shortcuts, but if you focus on BUILDING with the right mindset, vision, and hard work, you can reach all your goals. I have created a life that I love. I am constantly improving and learning. It never ends, but it's never boring.

In a world of convenience and noise, choose the harder path, and you will find peace and stillness. I promise it's worth it. The benefits of choosing to climb, and staying in that ascension mentality, are exponential when it comes to your mental and physical health. Trust me. The more you commit to your growth process, the more energy, stamina, clarity, happiness, organization, and concentrated attention will come your way. This brings your vision into focus.

The only caveat is--you have to be in it for the long game and trust that healing and change take time. You have the power to do it.

PART 3
BUSINESS

In life, you have two choices:

1) Try new things and get out of your comfort zone.

2) Keep things the way that they are.

Ask yourself, "What is the biggest, juiciest dream I have for my life? The biggest, baddest goal, no matter how ridiculous it may seem?" Take note of your answers, and then work backward from there. Reverse engineer it.

Do you know what I did with my life? I turned it on its head.

I've created three fully functioning and thriving businesses. No, it hasn't been easy.

When it comes to business, you have to OWN your power and get ready to work. Figure out what you're passionate about, what you're good at, and what you're not good at. Be honest with yourself about the time, finances, and effort it will take for you to get to where you want to go and aim high. Then, chew on this . . .

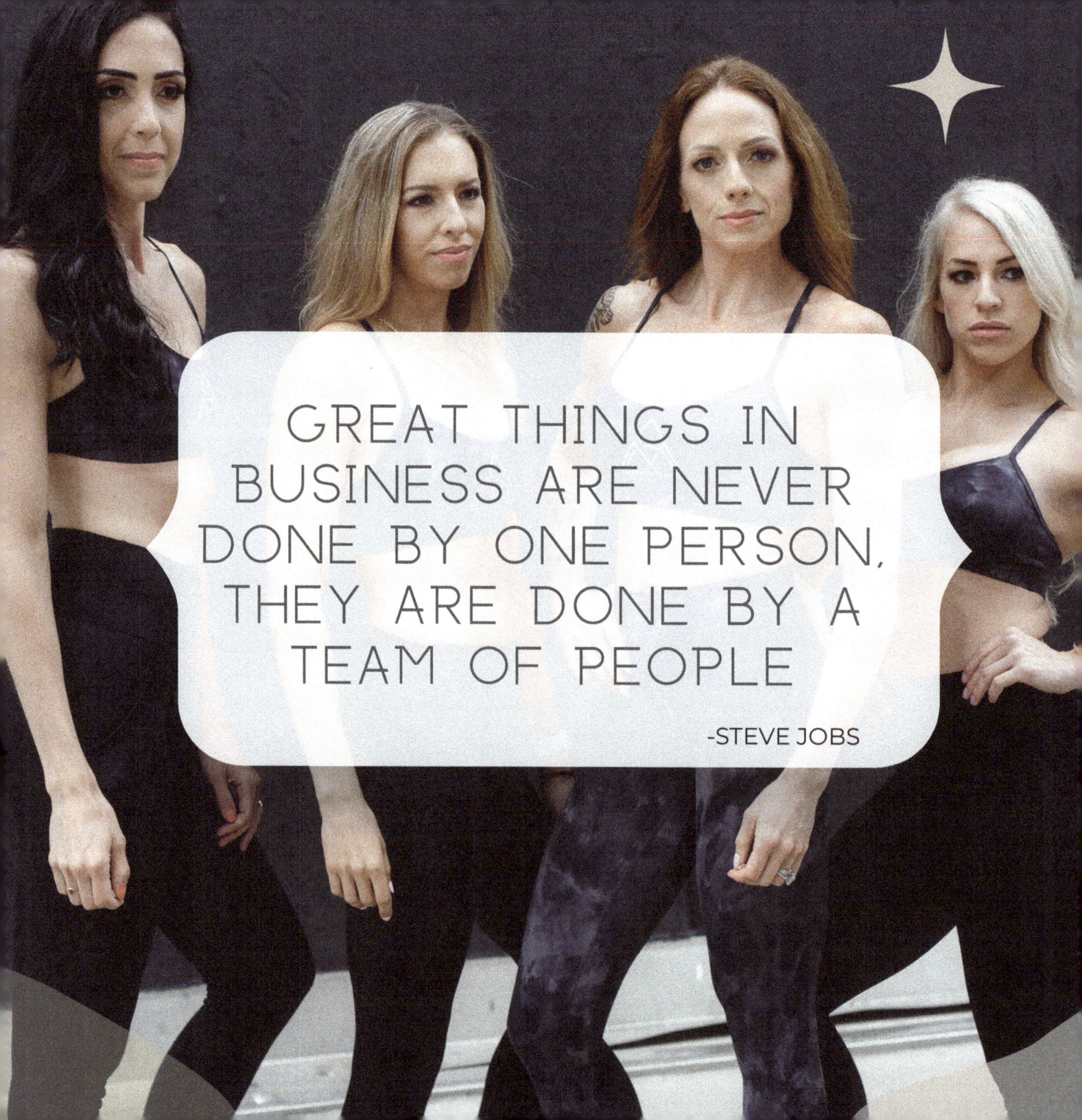

YOUR TEAM MATTERS

Business is not solely based on what you provide for your clients, but what you provide for yourself and your team as well, in order to create a culture of wellness. Knowing your capabilities, start by setting priorities for yourself and your team. Having the foundation of a structured day with enough free space in between is essential to give yourself the creative freedom to let the flow happen.

Choosing the people that will be by your side in your business is key. I have strategically recruited and hired a powerful team that aligns with my values and goals. They know I have their back, and they have mine. My businesses are set up to help and serve others. Our teams' well-being and work-life balance matters and allows us to be present and give our all to our clients. It begins in house.

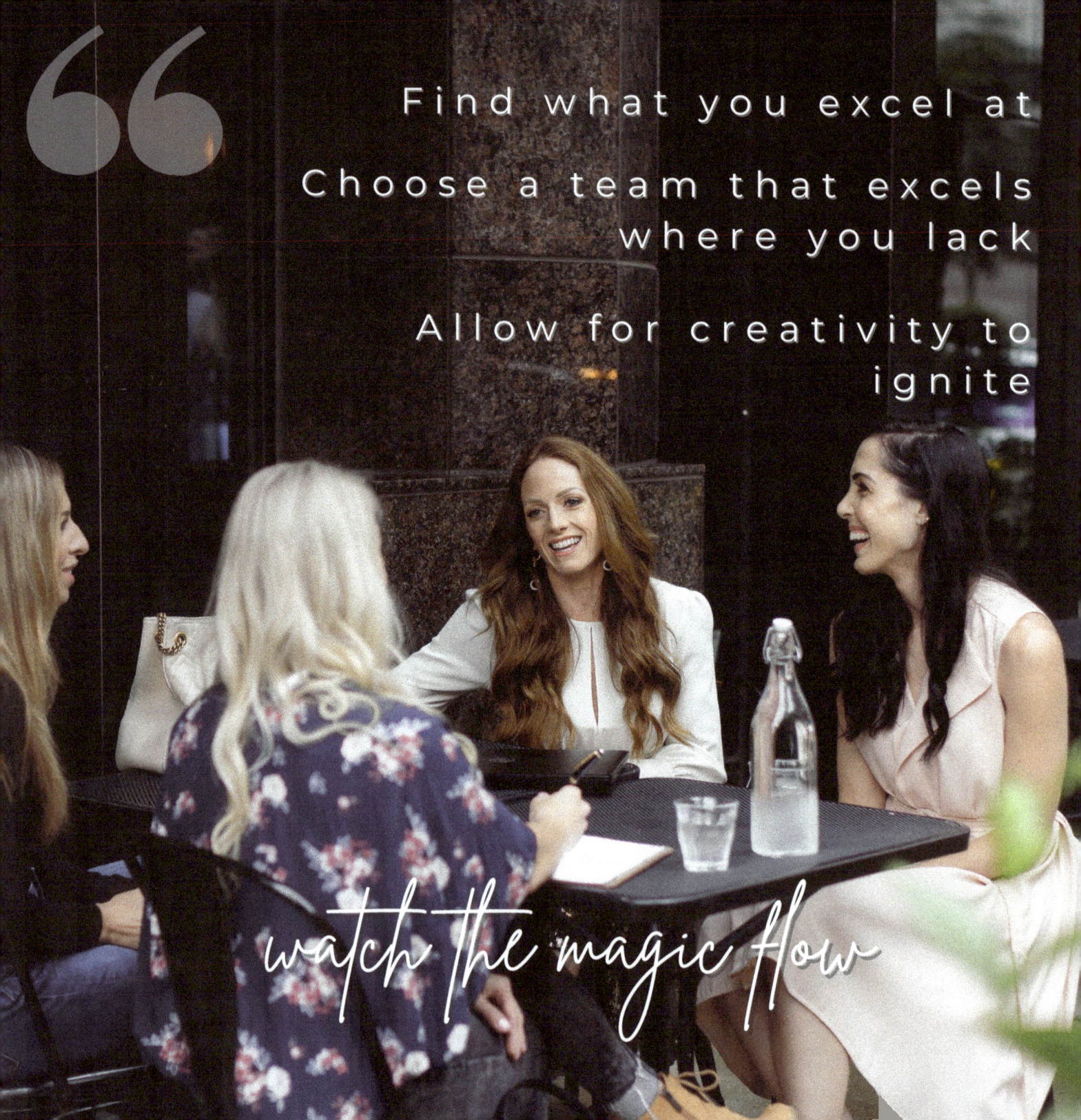

DELEGATE & EXECUTE

In business, it's necessary sometimes to take a step back and reevaluate your processes. What needs to be accomplished first? What can you delegate to your team so that you have more free time to focus on more important items? What can YOU accomplish in that free time? I farm out what I am not good at or what is NOT a valuable way to spend my time. I have an admin and a marketing team. I've learned the power of delegation.

While it's important to delegate tasks to your team, it's crucial to give them the space to unlock their OWN creative process. I developed processes that allow my business to run smoothly, and I rely on those systems. I stay out of the way of my employees' process.

Be aware of this: your employees' time is just as valuable as yours, and you must treat it that way. Just as my own creative process and content creation is the most important part of my workday, whatever they're passionate about--that is part of their ascension process--is honored and has a place. I want them to live healthy and thriving lives so that their time at work is well spent. Our work and passions take precedence over mundane tasks--it's our NON-NEGOTIABLE. It should be yours, too.

> "Surround yourself with emotionally healthy people. OR ones that are striving to become healthier."

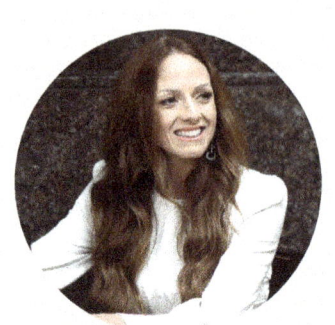

AMY WILHELMI

MENTAL HEALTH THERAPIST, ENTREPRENEUR, SPEAKER, ATHLETE

RELATIONSHIPS.
RELATIONSHIPS.
RELATIONSHIPS.

All my businesses are different yet similar. All of them involve people and are relationship-oriented. I value community and relationships over the bottom line, and both clients and employees feel this. When I give to my community and work hard at establishing relationships, the business grows organically.

This should be the basis for all businesses. For them to flow efficiently but naturally, there must be an essence of creative freedom that is structured enough to ensure the needs of clients and the business itself are met.

In my experience, putting people first and actively listening to understand them has made all the difference. Now that I'm on the other side—helping others build and scale their own lives—I see more than ever that it's all about your tribe. My passion has taken a turn to helping business owners get there and find their people, too.

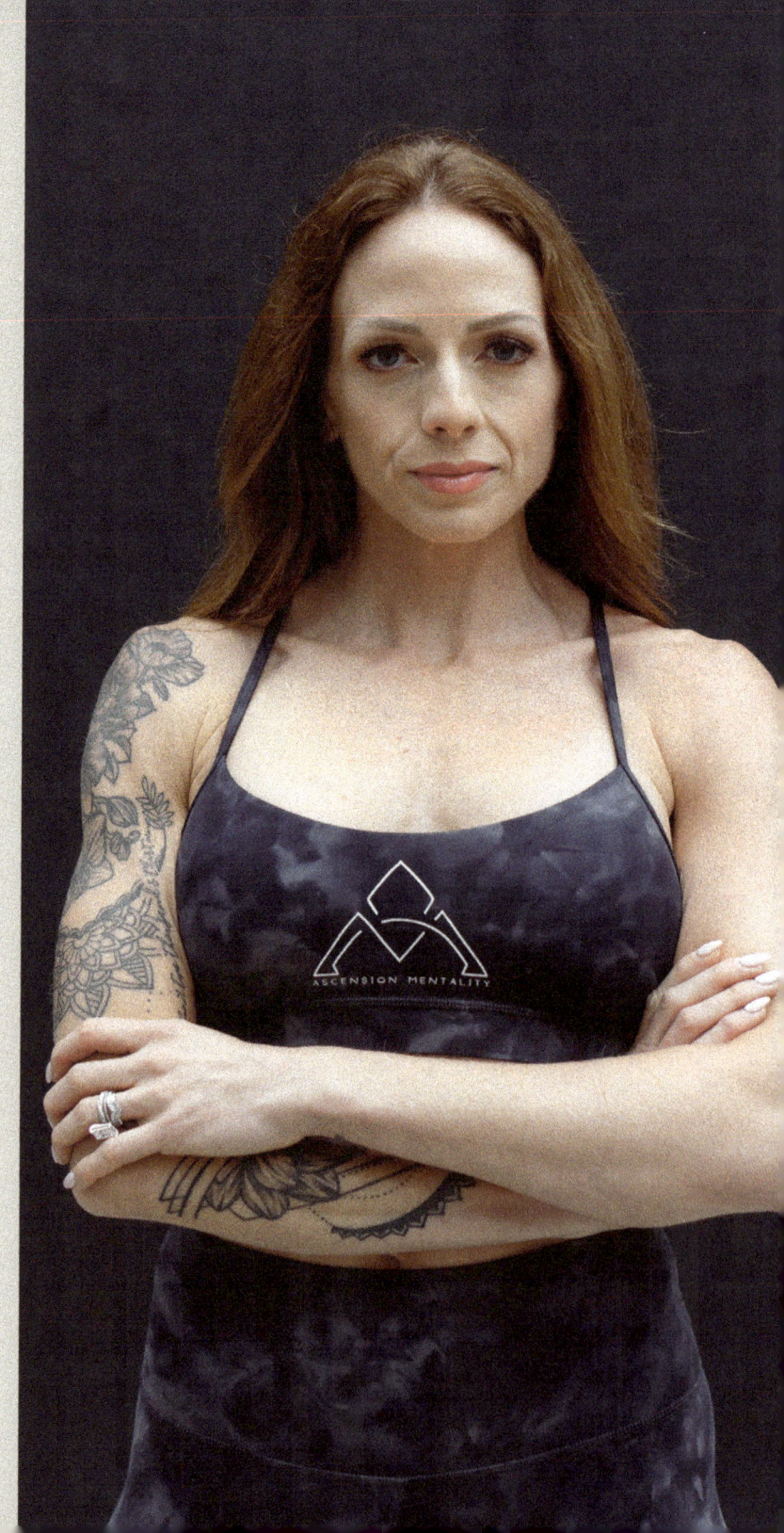

> "VISUALIZE YOUR HIGHEST SELF AND START SHOWING UP AS HER"

KEEP YOUR EYES ON THE PRIZE

Remember that belief system we talked about? It applies to everything--your money, your growth, and your business. Living in that abundance mindset will propel you to keep reaching new heights.

I think about one time when I was in a hotel room on vacation with my kids. I signed the contract for my 16-room business office space. I said YES. I jumped in. I had no idea what was truly coming, but I knew that it had to be a success. I had to figure it out. I closed my eyes and envisioned what I wanted my life to look like. I didn't know what the journey would hold, but I knew what kind of life I wanted.

Fast forward six years and l did figure it out. Hard work brought me here. My ascension mentality brought me here. In any goal you have, you must be able to visualize the end result, and that's probably not even big enough. If you asked me then if I'd be here today, writing this to you, I hadn't dreamt big enough yet.

Don't get swayed or distracted. Keep your eyes on that prize. Today, I'm passionate about leading by example and showing business owners or potential business owners that they CAN do it all. There's no competition but yourself. If I can do it, you can do it.

After all, the only ceiling is in your mind. Go get it!

MANIFESTO

I believe in mental fortitude. I believe in the universe of possibilities that lies inside each of us to heal, level up, and live our best life. I believe in people's ability to not only survive but to thrive. I believe in the power of connection. I believe in raw, transparent, truth-telling storytelling. I believe in people's innate ability to be resilient, to overcome challenges, and come out on the other side with mental wellness.

I BELIEVE IN OUR COLLECTIVE HUMAN TRIBE.

#MentalHealthRocks #MentalFormula #ThePoweroftheMind #HumanTribe #MindFormula #MindsetWorld #AscensionMentality #AmyWilhelmi #MakeMentalGains

ABOUT THE AUTHOR

Amy believes in the power of mental fortitude and the many possibilities that lie inside individuals to level up and live their best lives. Within her work, Amy encourages the power of connection and the development of raw, transparent, and truth-telling storytelling. Amy sees people's innate abilities to be resilient and overcome challenges through mental wellness tools and techniques.

By sharing her personal story of being a business owner, licensed marriage and family therapist, divorce mediator, performance coach, mother, and bikini bodybuilder, Amy hopes to make a difference in the lives of others. She encourages people to let go of judgment, stigma, shame, and self-consciousness so they step into their own truths and powers and feel relieved, relaxed, and ready to conquer life.

For more information about Amy Wilhelmi, visit:
www.amywilhelmi.com

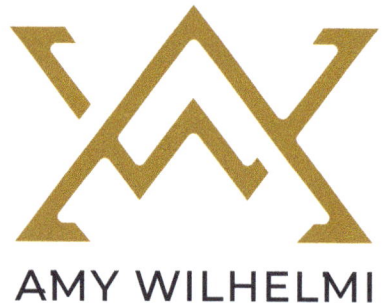

www.ingramcontent.com/pod-product-compliance
Lightning Source LLC
Chambersburg PA
CBHW040021300426
43673CB00107B/337